CLINICAL PRESCRIBER TO INDIAN MOTHER TINCTURES

New Weapon In The Armoury

NITESH JAIN, M.D.

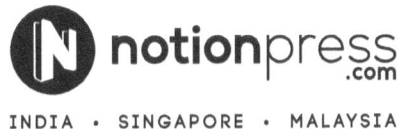

INDIA • SINGAPORE • MALAYSIA

Notion Press Media Pvt Ltd

No. 50, Chettiyar Agaram Main Road,
Vanagaram, Chennai, Tamil Nadu – 600 095

First Published by Notion Press 2021
Copyright © Nitesh Jain, M.D. 2021
All Rights Reserved.

ISBN 978-1-63957-442-1

This book has been published with all efforts taken to make the material error-free after the consent of the author. However, the author and the publisher do not assume and hereby disclaim any liability to any party for any loss, damage, or disruption caused by errors or omissions, whether such errors or omissions result from negligence, accident, or any other cause.

While every effort has been made to avoid any mistake or omission, this publication is being sold on the condition and understanding that neither the author nor the publishers or printers would be liable in any manner to any person by reason of any mistake or omission in this publication or for any action taken or omitted to be taken or advice rendered or accepted on the basis of this work. For any defect in printing or binding the publishers will be liable only to replace the defective copy by another copy of this work then available.

CONTENTS

Preface .... *v*

Introduction .... *xv*

List of Medicine and Abbreviation .... *xxiii*

1. Clinical Prescriber 1
2. Repertory of Investigations 21
3. Caution 27
4. Mode of Preparation of Homoeopathic Mother Tinctures of Plant Kingdom 31
5. List of Plants with Its Part Used for Preparation of Mother Tincture 36
6. List of Medicines with Their Common Names in Sanskrit and Hindi 44

PREFACE

Ayurved, the treatment of Indian sub-continent is been practiced since ages. Generally they use crude form of drug basing on their concept of balancing "Baat", "Pitt", and "Kauf" to attain health. Materia Medica of Ayurved called "Dravyagun Shastra" mentions action of drug in broad and crude way unlike Homoeopathic Materia Medica. So we see that many uses of Indian mother tinctures matches with their Ayurved counterparts but many do not match. As, when mother tincture is made of a mother substance it differs from the crude substance in all forms, thereby its action differs.

My interest in mother tinctures arose when during my 1st proff. in Kumaoun University I saw Prof. (Dr.) H. S. Chouhan our H. O. D. of Physiology to prescribe Raoulfia serpentina Q and Berberis vulgaris Q in 20 gtt dose every 15 min to a patient of malignant hypertension. Being neophyte I asked him his reason of prescription. He humbly told that Raoulfia will reduce the function of heart and Berberis will increase function of kidneys thereby if patient urinates after the dose then it implies that his condition is being taken to the path of recovery. This physiological concept in therapeutics made deep impression and bent my mind towards such physiological doses.

As time passed, in 3rd proff. I came in contact with our Assoc. Prof. (Dr.) P. S. Kumar, from Dept. of Organon of Medicine. He used to prepare indigenous mother tinctures and use it in various types of cases in college O. P. D. This turned my mind towards Indian Mother Tinctures and I gradually started to use it in my practice.

Medicines should be made from genuine substances and mode of preparation should be as mentioned in pharmacopeia. But, in reality we come across different results in same medicine of different companies. More worse same mother tincture of different companies are of different colour, consistency and smell; this shows that somewhere difference is present either in collection of mother substance or in manufacturing it. To decrease this ambiguity and have reliable medicines Hahnemann asked physician to prepare his own medicines.

"Substances which are indigenous to a particular area are best suited to ailments occurring to organism in that particular environment." We see this to come true in clinical practice. On talking about this with my junior Dr. Amit Vohra, he opined that work on tinctures will be helpful for newcomers to gain confidence in Homoeopathy. Newcomers are confused in selection of medicines and if it is selected then greater confusion occurs in respect to its doses and repetition. Thereby, I took up the task to make a Clinical Prescriber of Indian Mother Tinctures from experience including posology wherever possible.

All said and done, I have to take permission of my Mentor Prof. (Dr.) H. S. Rath. I was scared to ask him as this is not the aim of Homoeopathic therapeutics – to palliate, but I use it in practice and get good results in numerous cases so, asked him with courage. To my surprise he did not scold me rather encouraged me to do such work as it is the need of the day and agreed to write an "Introduction" to this work. My heart is greatly moved by his act and I thank him for spending his valuable time for writing such an amazing Introduction.

Protocol Used to Prepare Repertory

Majority of physicians using mother tinctures in practice use it in conjuction with potentized medicine or in combination of tinctures. So in order to know pure effect of tinctures only those cases in which the tincture is used singly without any potentized medicine or any other adjuvant like mother tinctures or biochemics etc. are selected. Retrospective study of these cases showed efficacy of particular tincture in particular condition. So, only those conditions were picked up and mentioned in the form of rubric and medicine is indicated. After seeing numerous cases we come to conclusion that particular medicine acts best in particular doses and repetition. To reach this point needs much effort, time and experience with a deep insight into the case. So, wherever any particular dose is seen to be much effective it is mentioned. Rest is left for further experience.

Being a clinician many a times I came across conditions in which I was left with only reports of Investigations and nothing else to prescribe on. This led me to ponder over and do some work in this aspect. Gradually I had collected some data of few medicines and put it in form of rubrics of investigations. Hope in near future many Physicians will come forward and give addition of their experience to this work and make it more complete one.

In this work those medicines which are well proved and present in Materia Medica is not mentioned like –

1. Anacardium occidentale.
2. Anacardium orientale.
3. Coculus indica.
4. Nux moschata.
5. Nux vomica.

6. Nyctanthes arbortristis.

7. Plantago major.

8. Zingiber officinalis.

Some Indian medicines could not be used due to non availability of patients like –

1. Berberis aristata.

2. Calotropis lactum.

3. Curcuma caesia.

4. Curcuma zedoaria.

5. Granatum.

6. Luffa amara.

7. Nymphoea odorata.

8. Sewrtia chiraita.

Many more Indian medicines used in Ayurved since ages is waiting to be used in tincture form in Homoeopathy, as time passes I will try to use them and put forward my experience in this regard, to the profession.

Arrangement of the Prescriber

In this prescriber at the onset the list of medicine along with their abbreviation is mentioned, followed by the text containing the clinical rubrics, no major differentiation is mentioned in the sub rubrics as it is a handy bed side prescriber so mostly the rubrics that we come across in clinic is mentioned along with the medicine in short form.

Wherever the condition is seen numerous times and its dose is confirmed it is mentioned. This is the dose that I came across by experience and found to be true. Wherever many patients are not seen or doses were fluctuating, no doses are mentioned. Then there are rubrics pertaining to common pathological investigations. This is mentioned to make the physician aware of the effect of medicines inside the body.

There are many instances where medicines are not available in market so brief mode of preparation of medicines is mentioned by using which a physician can make use of his own prepared medicines at the hour of need, in the interest of the patient followed by a section on "Caution" for caution to be taken while using a particular drug.

While writing it, a thought flashed in mind that many will not know the botanical names of the species so to overcome this at last the common names of the plant is mentioned in vernacular languages, still many names could not be known so it is left for further editions.

When to use Mother Tinctures

After all the work, it becomes necessary to know that under which circumstances we need to employ mother tinctures. As we know that all substance have its dynamicity, which is increased by potentization, this means that mother tinctures too have dynamicity; of course too less, but it can be used as supportive measure in following cases –

1. In cases where physiological action of medicine is required. Researches shows that Beta vulgaris slows down the action of heart causing hypotension.

2. In beginning of any problem when it is at superficial level. Initially if anyone suffers from cold Allium cepa restores his health quickly.

3. In treatment of chronic diseases when any deep acting anti miasmatic medicine is employed and any acute problem arise, then mother tincture can be used, without hampering the action of already employed medicine. Like older individuals undergoing any chronic treatment suffers from diarrhoea then Aegle marmelos quickly takes care of his bowel.

4. In cases which requires palliation due to advanced pathology. This is mostly seen in advance cases of carcinoma where metastasis has taken place and much dark, offensive bleeding occurs, to arrest it Cinnamonum is useful.

5. In old age, trivial symptoms can be well managed by mother tinctures, then better to avoid potentized medicines. Very often we find sleeplessness with weak memory in old age, this condition can be easily tackled by Bacopa munneri.

6. In cases where medicine is not indicated, mother tinctures can be used to give relief in some problem of patient and gain his confidence. At times in emergency we see that patient is bleeding profusely then we have to arrest bleeding to save him from hypovolumia; Blumea odorata works miraculously here.

7. In those cases which come after much palliation from dominant school of medicine, then mother tincture shall be used to counteract the withdrawal symptoms. Mostly in psychiatric cases where the patient is under treatment for decades, when he is given Acorus calamus he easily comes out of effects of previously taken medicines.

8. Whenever the patient is in addiction for long time then mother tincture counteracts his withdrawal symptoms. Aven sat counteracts the effect of opium addiction.

9. In cases where immediate relief is needed and experience proves that mother tincture never fails to give results. When we see that indicated Sulphur is not working up to expectation and burning is still present in patient's body then Semal acts. This I say from experience.

Way to use this Clinical Prescriber

Selecting any problem of the case in hand, on seeing this work we see that only basic clinical rubrics are mentioned which we generally come across in clinics. To familiarize with this work I ask you to go through the work at least once in a month initially so that it becomes handy for use at time of need. Some points to be kept in mind while using this work -

1. Along with the indicated medicine in a rubric, wherever doses and repetition is confirmed; it is mentioned, else only short form of medicine is mentioned.

2. List of medicine along with its abbreviation is mentioned at the onset of the book.

3. In this prescriber where no potency is mentioned use Mother tincture, but wherever any other lower potency is found to be acting better than mother tincture then it is indicated.

4. Where ever nothing is mentioned regarding use of water use normal water, wherever experience showed that taking medicine in warm water is beneficial, it is mentioned.

Preface

5. After the medicine is selected, section "Caution" should be consulted to see the contraindications if any and proceed likewise.

6. Meanings of short forms used –
   - Gtt ⇒ Drops.
   - OD ⇒ Once a day.
   - BD ⇒ Twice a day.
   - SOS ⇒ Take when required.
   - TDS ⇒ Thrice a day.
   - H_2O ⇒ Water.

List of Contributors

While I apparently completed this work I thought that it is very difficult to use all the medicines in all types of patients where it is applicable. So I shall add experiences of other physicians and I began to contact them; but I could not succeed to gain their knowledge and put forward to the profession. Only a few agreed to share their experiences. So, I added experiences of following persons in this work. Additions have their codes at the end. These are the names of those persons without whom the work would not have taken this form.

1. Dr. Priya Shankar Kumar, B.Sc. B.H.M.S. (psk).

   Former, Assoc. Prof. C. H. Medical college and Hospital, Rudrapur.

2. Dr. Abhishekh Trivedi, BSc, BHMS, ND. (at).

   Advance Homoeo Care, Rai Barely.

3. Dr. Sumit Kumar Chauhan, M.D. (skc)

    Asst. Prof. C. H. Medical college and Hospital, Rudrapur.

4. Dr. Bharati Tripathy, M.D. (Scholar), (bt)

    F. D. H. Medical college and Hospital. Aurangabad.

I ask all the members of Fraternity using Indian Mother Tinctures in practice to open up and give your additions which will be added in next edition with your name.

This Clinical Prescriber would not see the light of the day without the constant effort of Notion Press, Nikitha Lalwani, Yeshwini Doshi, and Urmi Mukherjee. Lastly, special thanks to Mrs. Abha Garg for her typing in Sanskrit and Hindi.

Finally thanks goes to my patients who kept their faith in me and Homoeopathy rendering my perception to be much clearer.

My attempt here is virgin so, mistakes are mandatory, corrections and suggestions are solicited.

Vapi, Gujarat. Nitesh Jain
15th May, 2021. drniteshhomoeopath@gmail.com

INTRODUCTION

The selection of right remedy is one of the herculean tasks before a genuine homoeopathic physician, who works for the weal of suffering mankind. The administration of remedy in proper dose and its repetition requires a good deal of reflection.

In the initial phase of progress of Homoeopathy when the number of proved medicines was meagre, the selection of remedy was easy although the perfectly suitable remedy was hardly available for each and every case of disease out of the limited treasure. The volume of positive symptoms of medicines on human beings went on increasing in due course of drug proving by Hahnemann. It became a difficult task to grasp all the symptoms of all medicines in mind. Thus, there appeared the need for quick reference of medicines against symptoms. To compliment this need, in the year 1805 he published the book "Fragmenta de viribus medicamentorum positivis, sive in sano corpore humano observatis". First part of this book contains the proved symptoms and the second part, index to symptoms indicating medicines. This second part is a repertory that finds its origin in the field of Homoeopathy. Thereafter his faithful follower, Dr. C. M. F. Von Boenninghausen and several others did tremendous development in the field of repertory. While writing the second edition of "The Theory of Chronic Diseases their Peculiar Nature and their Homoeopathic Cure" in 1838 he has mentioned that a physician while selecting remedy not to be satisfied with any of the existing repertories for these books are only intended to give light hints as to one or other remedy that might be selected, but they can never dispense him from making the research at the first fountain head. The volume of Materia Medica by this time has become so much bulky that the means of easy reference has become inevitable. Thus, there has developed the several soft-wares besides the voluminous books on repertory to provide the hints towards remedy selection although the final selection of remedy must be left up to the judgment of the physician after a critical analysis and thorough study to each case from several dimensions.

In the preface to the fifth volume of the second edition of "The Theory of Chronic Diseases their Peculiar Nature and their Homoeopathic Cure" in 1838 he has mentioned that the modern homoeopathic physicians were hesitating the use of medicines even of thirtieth potency. They were using lower potencies having less developed medicinal virtue in more massive preparations in larger doses. So, they were unable to accomplish what the art of Homoeopathy can do. He has mentioned further that every minute pellet moistened with medicine at fiftieth potency dissolved in a quantity of water and taken in small parts little produce violent action with sensitive patients. Such a preparation contains almost all the properties latent in the drug now fully developed, and these can only then come into full activity.

No doubt medicines selected on the basis of greater matching of characteristic symptoms of the patient with that of medicine, and administered in minimum dose in high potency bring forth more beneficial result than those selected on the basis of common symptoms and administered in low potency and massive doses. This is the basic concept of genuine as well as ideal practice in Homoeopathy. The cases not mismanaged with large doses of medicine of any system, nor gone to the irreversible pathological changes, nor having several obstacles to cure are very nicely managed by such treatment in an ideal way. But, in real practice such ideal cases coming to the physician directly are less in number. A physician has to deal with several varieties of cases many of which are difficult to handle.

It is instructed that when a patient comes from other physician after taking much medicine, the physician has to wait by giving placebo till the effect of already taken medicines is over, after which he has to administer the suitable remedy on the basis of fresh collection of symptoms of the patient. Such ideal instruction is difficult to follow in some situations where patient is accustomed with taking large doses of palliative medicines like sedative, anti-hypertensive, anti-diabetic, analgesics, etc. In some such cases a severe secondary action, counter action is not observed after stopping such medicines where as in some other cases such counter action is prominently marked that obliges the patient to discontinue placebo and take recourse of previously continued palliatives. A homoeopathic physician, who has to earn his bread and butter from the profession, searches an immediate palliative measure to somehow manage the case by administration of mother tinctures at his stock before handling cautiously to prepare it for genuine Homoeopathic treatment with Similimum in high potency and minimum dose.

There are certain irreversible pathological conditions like some endocrinal disorders, genetic disorders, etc, which can hardly return to normalcy and almost require life-long palliation. Consequently, if a Homoeopathic physician after his sincere effort to bring radical cure through the genuine practice fails to achieve his goal, he may manage such cases with palliative means through administration of mother tincture.

At certain occasions the condition of the patient becomes so weak or exhausted that it becomes difficult to bring a reaction in the human organism by the help of potentised homoeopathic medicines that require sufficient energy to overcome the action of remedy in secondary action, curative action. Such cases need immediate palliation. E.g., Severe anaemia resulting from excessive haemorrhage from haemorrhoids or from uterus, sudden unconsciousness, etc. The genuine Homoeopathic treatment with similimum in suitable potency and minimum dose becomes possible only after the severe acute condition is somehow temporarily managed by some mother tincture.

Homoeopathic practice is based on strict individualisation unlike routinism prevailing in allopathy. The art of healing in Homoeopathy requires genius physicians, the number of which is actually less in this field. It is out of the reason that the palliative treatment prevailing in allopathy, yielding quick relief, draws attention of public. Accordingly, the majority of intelligent medical professionals are attracted towards allopathy and become a part of that profession. On the other hand, Homoeopathy that renders radical cure in time consuming way is able to attract less numbers of intelligent mass. Still then there are some intelligent allopathic doctors, who are converted to Homoeopathy by realizing its efficacy in the cure of chronic diseases and consequently preventing the acute diseases. Thus, a significant number of Homoeopathic physicians are less able for optimal utilization of their skill in selection of Similimum and poor in knowledge as well as experience. Such Homoeopathic physicians if find difficulty on their part for genuine Homoeopathic practice in a safe way, they may use mother tinctures having little toxic effect, as well as low potency, general store medicines instead of using deep acting anti-miasmatic medicines, which are not free from harm when administered in high potency and in large doses.

Introduction

It is a tendency of patients to expect quick improvement since the beginning of Homoeopathic treatment. Although such improvement becomes possible by suitable Homoeopathic treatment by experienced Homoeopathic Physicians in acute diseases, it is less expected in chronic diseases. But, the experienced Physician doing practice since long and who has gained the faith of people while advices patient to wait for improvement in chronic diseases then many people wait and continue treatment. But, this is hardly the case with neophyte having less experience and less faith of public upon them. Such neophytes while handling cases of chronic diseases of long standing in the patients, who become impatient for quick relief, may administer harmless mother tinctures to bring certain improvement. Later on, when the patient gains some confidence upon him, he may discontinue the use of mother tincture and manage with proper Homoeopathic treatment in genuine manner.

Indigenous medicines are more valuable than those imported from foreign countries out of the reason that these are available at low price due to less expense on transportation and low tax. The purity of medicine relating to its genuineness is essential for optimal action. Sometimes it comes to notice that the same mother tincture purchased from different companies are available in different colours. The reason behind it is that they do not utilise the exact species of the concerned genus or they do not utilise the exact part of the original drug substance or secretion or excretion required for the purpose. Thus, the advantage of indigenous drug substance is that a Homoeopathic physician can prepare medicine by his own for his practice by taking the pure drug substance and its required part available in his locality which is difficult to collect for medicines prepared from utilising those from foreign countries. Besides this, medicines available in the locality where a person lives are provided by nature for his protection and according to the need of the geographical situation. E.g., Human beings in hot summer are liable to dehydration and reduced output of urine. Watermelon providing water and at the same time acting as a diuretic is available in India in summer season that satisfies the need of body for water and helps in increasing urine output.

After going through the above stated instructions an experienced and genuine Homoeopathic physician must not be swayed from the right path of treatment in ideal manner. He may use the palliative measures only exceptionally either when his capability to handle any particular case in genuine way is inadequate or while the situation with the patient compels him to adopt such measure. A beginner may work cautiously to gain the confidence of patients through the application of his knowledge and means according to situations and try to rectify his work towards perfection throughout his professional carrier.

Dr. Nitesh Jain, a sincere, honest and dedicated physician in the field of Homoeopathy has taken immense pain in procuring the indigenous mother tinctures in as pure form as possible. He has applied these in suitable dose on different patients suffering from different ailments and observed their effect. The effect of some new medicines, which were not proved earlier, is also observed by him through clinical application. He has not only written it in the form of indicating medicine in "Prescriber" but also has mentioned the dose and its repetition schedule, which is a complete work in helping the Physician to use the indicated medicine without ambiguity. The medicines indicated against "Chronic fatigue syndrome" can be used at the first sight without a greater analysis. In this prescriber the section on "Diseases and conditions" lists medicines which can be employed in those circumstances where nothing is clearly indicated. Section on "Concomitant" is useful

Introduction

where particular concomitant is clear and marked without any other symptom. This surely ameliorates the problem of the patient. His basic object is to transfer his knowledge and experience to the profession at the greater interest of suffering humanity. His mission would be fulfilled if the Physicians would apply the knowledge propagated through this literature is applied in practice as per the exact guideline and thereby rendering immense benefit to mankind.

Kashipur, UK.

May 17th, 2021.   Himanshu Shekhar Rath.

LIST OF MEDICINE AND ABBREVIATION

Sl.No.	List of Medicine.	Abbreviation.
1.	Abelmoschus moschatus.	Abel mos.
2.	Abroma augusta.	Abro aug.
3.	Abroma radix.	Abro rad.
4.	Abrus precatorius.	Abr pre.
5.	Acalypha indica.	Aca ind.
6.	Achyranthes aspera.	Ach asp.
7.	Acorus calamus.	Aco cal.
8.	Aegle folia.	Aeg fol.
9.	Aegle marmelos.	Aeg mar.
10.	Agnus cas.	Agn cas.
11.	Allium cepa.	All cep.
12.	Allium sativa.	All sat.
13.	Aloe vera.	Alo ver.
14.	Amoora rohituka.	Ammo roh.

List of Medicine and Abbreviation

Sl.No.	List of Medicine.	Abbreviation.
15.	Amygdala amara.	Amy am.
16.	Ananas sativa.	Ana sat.
17.	Andersonia rohitika.	And roh.
18.	Andrographis paniculata.	And pan.
19.	Arctium lappa.	Arc lap.
20.	Areca catechu.	Are cat.
21.	Aristolochia indica.	Arist ind.
22.	Asai.	Asai.
23.	Asafoetida.	Asaf.
24.	Atista indica.	Atis ind.
25.	Atista radix.	Atis rad.
26.	Avena sativa.	Aven sat.
27.	Averrhoa bilimbi.	Aver bi.
28.	Azadirachta indica.	Aza ind.
29.	Bacopa munneri.	Bac mun.
30.	Beta vulgaris.	Bet vul.
31.	Bauhinia variegate.	Bau var.
32.	Blatta orientalis.	Blat ori.
33.	Blumea odorata.	Blu od.
34.	Boerhaavia diffusa.	Boe diff.

Sl.No.	List of Medicine.	Abbreviation.
35.	Boerhaavia repens.	Boe rep.
36.	Caesalpinia bonducella.	Caes bon.
37.	Calendula officinalis.	Calen off.
38.	Calotropis gigentea.	Cal gig.
39.	Cannabis indica.	Can ind.
40.	Cannabis sativa.	Can sat.
41.	Cantharanthus roseus.	Cant ros.
42.	Carica papaya.	Car pap.
43.	Carum carvi.	Car car.
44.	Cassia fistula.	Cas fist.
45.	Cassia sophera.	Cas sop
46.	Catalpa bignonioides.	Cat big.
47.	Cephalendra indica.	Cep ind.
48.	Chrysopogon zizanioides.	Chry zin.
49.	Cinnamonum.	Cinna.
50.	Citrus limonum.	Cit lim.
51.	Clerodendron infortunatum.	Cler inf.
52.	Coccus cacti.	Cocc cac.
53.	Coleous aromaticus.	Col aro.
54.	Coriandrum sativum.	Cor sat.

List of Medicine and Abbreviation

Sl.No.	List of Medicine.	Abbreviation.
55.	Crateva nurvala.	Crat nur.
56.	Crocus sativa.	Cro sat.
57.	Croton tig.	Crot t.
58.	Cucurbita pepo.	Cuc pep.
59.	Cuminum cyminum.	Cum cym.
60.	Curcuma longa.	Cur lon.
61.	Cynodon dactylon.	Cyn dac.
62.	Cyperus rotundus.	Cyp rot.
63.	Cyperus scariosus.	Cyp sca.
64.	Daphne indica.	Daph ind.
65.	Daucus carota.	Dau car.
66.	Desmodium gangeticum.	Des gan.
67.	Dolichos lablab.	Doli lab.
68.	Eclipta alba.	Ecl alb.
69.	Embelia officinalis.	Emb off.
70.	Embelia ribes.	Emb rib.
71.	Ficus benghalensis.	Fic ben.
72.	Ficus indica.	Fic ind.
73.	Ficus religiosa.	Fic rel.
74.	Foeniculum vulgare.	Foe vul.

Sl.No.	List of Medicine.	Abbreviation.
75.	Genitsta tinctoria.	Gent tin.
76.	Gentiana chirata.	Gent chi.
77.	Glycyrrhiza glabra.	Gly gla.
78.	Guggulu.	Gug.
79.	Gymnema sylvestre.	Gym syl.
80.	Gynocordia odorata.	Gyno od.
81.	Hedra helix.	Hed hel.
82.	Helianthus annus.	Heli an.
83.	Hemidesmus indica.	Hemi ind.
84.	Hibiscus.	Hib.
85.	Holarrhena antidysentrica.	Hol ant.
86.	Hydrocotyle asiatica.	Hydr asia.
87.	Hygrophila spinosa.	Hygr spi.
88.	Janosia ashoka.	Jan ash.
89.	Juglans regia.	Jug reg.
90.	Justicea adhatoda.	Just ad.
91.	Justicea rubrum.	Just rub.
92.	Leukas aspera.	Leu as.
93.	Lobelia inflata.	Lob in.
94.	Luffa bindal.	Luf bin.

Sl.No.	List of Medicine.	Abbreviation.
95.	Mangifera indica.	Man ind.
96.	Makardhawj.	Mak.
97.	Menispernum.	Meni.
98.	Morus indica.	Mor ind.
99.	Nardostachys grandiflora.	Nar gf.
100.	Natrum mutiaticum bit.	Nat mur bit.
101.	Nyctanthis arbortristis.	Nyc arb.
102.	Ocimum basilicum.	Oci bas.
103.	Ocimum canum.	Oci can.
104.	Ocimum cariophylatum.	Oci car.
105.	Ocimum gratessium.	Oci grat.
106.	Ocimum radix.	Oci rad.
107.	Ocimum sanctum.	Oci san.
108.	Oldenlandia herbacea.	Old her.
109.	Oleum ricini.	Ole ric.
110.	Oleum santali.	Ole san.
111.	Opuntia vulgaris.	Op vul.
112.	Phyllanthus niruri.	Phy nir.
113.	Picrorhiza kurroa.	Pic kur.
114.	Piper nigrum.	Pip nig.

Sl.No.	List of Medicine.	Abbreviation.
115.	Psoralia corylifolia.	Psor cor.
116.	Rauvolfia serpentina.	Rau ser.
117.	Raphanus sativa.	Raph sat.
118.	Ricinus communis.	Ric com.
119.	Santalum album.	San alb.
120.	Sassurea lappa.	Sass lap.
121.	Semal.	Sem.
122.	Solonum nigrum.	Sol nig.
123.	Solanum xanthocarpus.	Sol xan.
124.	Stellaria media.	Stel med.
125.	Syzygium jambolinum.	Syz jam.
126.	Tephrosia purpurea.	Tep pur.
127.	Terminalia arjuna.	Term arj.
128.	Terminalia bellirica.	Term bel.
129.	Terminalia chebula.	Term che.
130.	Tinospora cordifolia.	Tin cor.
131.	Trachyspermum ammi.	Trac ammi.
132.	Tribulus terrestris.	Tri ter.
133.	Trichosanthes dioica	Tric dio.
134.	Tylophora indica.	Tyl ind.

Sl.No.	List of Medicine.	Abbreviation.
135.	Verbascum thapsus.	Verb tha.
136.	Veronia anthelminthica.	Ver ant.
137.	Viola odorata.	Vio od.
138.	Viola tricolor.	Vio tri.
139.	Viscum album.	Vis alb.
140.	Withania coagulans.	With coa.
141.	Withania somnifera.	With som.
142.	Withania somnifera folia.	With som fol.
143.	Withania somnifera rubra.	With som rub
144.	Wrightia tinctoria.	Wri tin.

CLINICAL PRESCRIBER

Injuries and Accidents
Bites

Honey bee (or other poisonous bee) ⇒ Ach asp. external application on site of bite.

Scorpion bite ⇒ Pic kur.

Unknown insect ⇒ Nat mur bit. external application on site of bite.

Fractures, to promote healing of bones ⇒ Term arj. 10 gtt x tds.

Haemorrhage

Active ⇒ Fic rel.

Bloody, bright red in morning and dark clotted in evening ⇒ Aca ind. 10 gtt x tds.

Passive ⇒ Man ind.

    Dark, thick, clots easily ⇒ Cro sat.

    Distension of abdomen, with ⇒ Aca ind.

Haemoptysis ⇒ Aca ind. 10 gtt x tds.

    Profuse ⇒ Just rub.

Idiopathic from mouth ⇒ Fic ind.

Injury from ⇒ Fic rel.

Offensive, cancer in ⇒ Cinna.

Any outlet, to stop ⇒ Blu od. 20 gtt x 15 min.

Gums, from ⇒ Man ind.

Haemorrhoids, from ⇒ Cyn dac. 20 gtt x 15 min.

Lungs, stomach, tuberculosis in ⇒ Aca ind.

Tooth extraction, after ⇒ Calen off. 20 gtt sos.

Laceration ⇒ Calen off. external application for dressing in ratio 1 : 5.

Suspended animation

Animal bite, from ⇒ Ach asp.

Breath, cannot take ⇒ Mak 1x. 5 gr x 15 min.

Body cold, as if about to die ⇒ Mak 1x. 5 gr x 15 min.

Scorpion bite ⇒ Leu as.

Aggravation

Heat ⇒ Hygr spi.

Appetite

Chronic intermittent fever in
    Decreased, ⇒ Leu as. 5 gtt x tds.

Decreased
    Dyspepsia, with ⇒ Tin cor.
    Increase, to ⇒ Emb off.

Increased
    Diabetes in ⇒ Abro aug. 10 gtt x tds.

Atrophy

⇒ With coa.

Muscles, paralysis progressive with ⇒ With som.

Seminal loss, due to ⇒ With som. 10 gtt x in warm H_2O x tds.

Blood pressure

Hypertension ⇒ Aco cal. 15 gtt x tds.
    Anxiety, with ⇒ Rau ser. 15 gtt x tds.
    Depression, with ⇒ Rau ser. 15 gtt x tds.
    Insomnia, with ⇒ Rau ser. 15 gtt x tds.
    Mental stress, due to ⇒ Rau ser. 15 gtt x tds.
    Obesity, with ⇒ All sat. 15 gtt x tds (psk)
    Systolic, to reduce, diastolic normal ⇒ Rau ser. 20 gtt x tds (at).

Hypotension, both systolic and diastolic towards lower side, increase to ⇒ Term arj. 10 gtt x tds.

Boils

Burst, to ⇒ Use Polutice of Cyn dac., Oci car.

Burning

Body Itching, with ⇒ Cas sop. 10 gtt x tds.

Summer in ⇒ Sem. 5 gtt x tds.

Urethra in, urination during and after ⇒ Can ind.

Calculi

Renal ⇒ Cas fist., Hemi ind.
    Aneuria, with ⇒ Col aro. 20 gtt x horis.
    Break to ⇒ Col aro. 15 gtt x tds.
    Pain with ⇒ Oci can. 10 gtt x tds.
    Vomiting, with ⇒ Oci can.

Cephalgia

Bile, increased with ⇒ Aza ind.
Cataract, with ⇒ Calo gig.
Dysmenorrhoea, with ⇒ Can ind.
Gastritis, with ⇒ Lob in.
Hypertensive ⇒ Jan ash. 3 gtt x od.
Unilateral ⇒ Jan ash.

Chronic fatigue syndrome

Anaemia due to ⇒ Hib. 5 gtt x tds in warm H_2O.
Blood loss, after ⇒ Cyn dact. 10 gtt x tds.
    Offensive, cancer in, after ⇒ Cinna.
Cephalgia with ⇒ Hydr asia.
Dysentery after ⇒ Hol ant. 10 gtt x tds.
Fever, acute after ⇒ Aven sat.
    Anorexia with ⇒ Leu as. 5 gtt x tds.
    Chronic in ⇒ Aven sat. 20 gtt x tds (skc).

Prolonged, after ⇒ And pan. 10 gtt x tds.

Repeated (Malaria), after ⇒ Tin cor.

General ⇒ With som. 20 gtt x tds.

Heart, problem, due to ⇒ Term arj, 10 gtt x tds.

Hypoglycemia, due to ⇒ Bet vul. 15 gtt x tds.

Leg weakness, with ⇒ Gent chi.

Leucorrhoea, after ⇒ Jan ash. 5 gtt x tds.

Before ⇒ Term arj.

Mascular fatigue ⇒ Jug reg.

Menses, profuse due to ⇒ Jan ash.

Blood red, red clot, keeps on oozing ⇒ Meni.

Mentally ⇒ Bac mun. 3 gtt x tds.

Physically, with ⇒ With som. 2 gtt x tds.

Narcotics overuse, after ⇒ Aven sat. 20 gtt x tds.

Physically (as if worked too much) ⇒ With som fol. 2 gtt x tds.

Seminal loss, after ⇒ With som. 20 gtt x tds.

Sexual intercourse, increased, due to, Females in ⇒ Aven sat. 20 gtt x tds.

Males in ⇒ With som. 20 gtt x tds.

Sleeplessness, after, old age in ⇒ Bac mun. 5 gtt x tds.

Trembling with ⇒ With som rub. 10 gtt x tds.

Tuberculosis after ⇒ Bet vul. 10 gtt x tds.

Urination, profuse after ⇒ Gym syl.

Uterine, problem, after ⇒ Jan ash. 10 gtt x tds.

Vital fluid loss, due to ⇒ Tin cor.

Writing, inable with ⇒ Cyn dac.

Concomitant

Anaemia with emaciation ⇒ Boe diff.

Aphonea ⇒ Sol xan.

Carcinoma ⇒ Hydr asia.

Cold, acute ⇒ Oci san.

    Chronic, catches cold easily ⇒ Luf bin.

Constipation ⇒ Term che. 20 gtt x tds.

Cough ⇒ Ole San.

Discharges Suppressed, due to ⇒ Lob in.

Dryness ⇒ Abro aug.

Dysmenorrhoea ⇒ Abro rad.

Dyspnoea ⇒ Term bel.

Fibromyalgia ⇒ Des gan.

    Fever, with ⇒ Hygr spi.

    Gastritis, with ⇒ With som fol. 2 gtt x tds.

Gastritis ⇒ Cep ind.

Gastro intestinal tract derangement ⇒ Emb off.

GORD ⇒ Abel mos.

Haemorrhage, bright red in morning and dark clotted in evening ⇒ Aca ind.

Icterus, infantile ⇒ And pan.

    Malaria, after ⇒ And pan.

Leucorrhoea ⇒ Jan ash. 5 gtt x tds.

Menses, Irregular ⇒ Jan ash. 5 gtt x tds.

    Scanty ⇒ Abro rad.

Nausea ⇒ Heli an.

Oedema ⇒ Aeg fol.

Oedema of upper & lower eyelids (in infants) ⇒ Aeg mar.

Pain, Navel around ⇒ Atis ind.
   Spleen in, defecation during ⇒ Asai.
      Urination during ⇒ Asai.
Palpitation, physical exertion increased when ⇒ Rau ser.
Perspiration, cold ⇒ Abr pre.
Psychic condition ⇒ With som.
Salivation, Profuse ⇒ Lob in.
Skin ailments, inveterate ⇒ Gyno od.
   Thick (Eczema, Lupus) ⇒ Hydr asia.
Sleepiness ⇒ Des gan.
Throat problem ⇒ Gargle in luke warm water with Term che. in ratio 1 : 4.
Urine, profuse ⇒ Syz jam.
Pungent ⇒ Emb rib.
Vaginal problem ⇒ Wash Vagina with lotion of Jan ash in ratio 1 : 9.
Vertigo ⇒ Term che.
Vomiting ⇒ Tin cor.

Cough, acute

Expectoration, Absent ⇒ Just ad. 10 gtt x tds.
   Aphonea, with ⇒ Aza ind., Sol xan.
   Dyspnoea, with ⇒ Cas sop.
Present, Dyspnoea, with ⇒ Blat ori. 20 gtt x 15 min.
Bloody, bright red in morning and dark clotted in evening ⇒ Aca ind.
Chronic, Expectoration, Absent, Dyspnoea, with ⇒ Cocc cac.

Diabetes mellitus

Allergy, chronic with ⇒ Hygr spin.
Burning, in body, with ⇒ Cep ind.
Carbuncle, with ⇒ Abro aug.
Diabetic cardiacmyopathy, with ⇒ Abro aug.
    Nephropathy, with ⇒ Abro aug.
    Neuropathy, with ⇒ Bac mun.
Dropsy, with ⇒ Cep ind.
Emaciation, with (esp. of waist) ⇒ Abro aug. 20 gtt x tds.
Erectile dysfunction, with ⇒ Gym syl. 15 gtt x tds.
Gastritis, with ⇒ Cep ind. 15 gtt x tds.
Icterus, with ⇒ Cep ind.
Reeling of head, Urination, profuse after ⇒ Cep ind.
Spermatorrhoea, with ⇒ Oci cari.
Sugar, in urine, to reduce ⇒ Syz jam. 20 gtt x tds.
Weakness, with ⇒ Abro aug.
Urination profuse after, ⇒ Gym syl.

Diseases and condition

Acne ⇒ Alo ver.
Anaemia ⇒ Cler inf.
    Emaciation, with ⇒ Boe diff.
    Oedema, with ⇒ Just ad.
Anorexia ⇒ Phy nir.
Aphonia, sudden ⇒ Sol xan.
Atherosclerosis ⇒ Gug.
Cancer ⇒ Cas fist.

Breast, of ⇒ Ammo roh.

Pancreas, of ⇒ Ammo roh.

Cholilithiasis ⇒ Cit lim, doses depending on weight of the patient x qid (psk).

Coryza, winters in ⇒ Bet vul. 10 gtt x tds (at).

Cystitis ⇒ Vio tri.

Depression ⇒ Cant ros.

Diabetes mellitus ⇒ Aver bi.

Dupytren's contracture ⇒ Arc lap.

Dyspnoea ⇒ Blat ori. 10 gtt. sos.

Dysmenorrhoea ⇒ Cyp sca.

Endometriosis ⇒ Vis alb.

G6PD deficiency anaemia ⇒ Aca ind.

Hydronephrosis ⇒ Boe diff. 10 gtt x tds (psk).

Hypotension ⇒ Term arj. 10 gtt x tds.

IBS ⇒ Cor sat. 10 gtt x tds.

Infertility, anovulation due to ⇒ Abr aug.

Impotency ⇒ Fic ben., With som. 10 gtt x tds. in luke warm water x 6 months.

Infection ⇒ Boe rep.

Insomnia ⇒ Nar gf.

Malaria ⇒ Gent chi.

Methemoglobinemia ⇒ Aca ind.

OA ⇒ Cur lon. 5 gtt x bd x 2 months. (bt)

Obesity, esp. abdomem, gluteal ⇒ Ach asp.

Palpitation ⇒ Aco cal.

PCOD ⇒ Jan ash. 20 gtt x od, skip during menses x 4 months. (bt)

PID ⇒ Jan ash. 20 gtt x tds (skc).

PMDD ⇒ Agn cas.

Priapism ⇒ Op vul.

Prolapse uterus, leucorrhoea with ⇒ Arc lap.

Psoriasis ⇒ Wri tin.

Arthritis, with ⇒ Stel med.

    RA ⇒ Tyl ind.

Rheumatism ⇒ Oci grat., Vio tri.

Ringworm ⇒ Hemi ind.

Sciatica ⇒ Gent tin.

Worm infestation ⇒ Hol ant. 5 gtt x tds. for weeks (bt).

Ear

Blowing sounds ⇒ Abro aug.

Ottorrhoea, tinitis with ⇒ Asai.

Eyes

Conjunctivitis ⇒ Abr pre.

Vision ⇒ Car car.

Face

Pimples ⇒ Chry ziz.

    Constipation, with ⇒ Term che.

    Small, red ⇒ Aza ind.

Itch violently ⇒ Syz jam.

Burning, intense with ⇒ Cas sop.

Fever

Anorexia with ⇒ And pan. 15 gtt x bd x 60 days (psk).

Before

    Burning, eyes in ⇒ Gent chi.

    Cold application, amel. ⇒ Caes bon.

    Cephalgia, temporal, throbbing pain ⇒ Caes bon.

During

    Thirst for cold water with moist tongue ⇒ Caes bon.

    Thirstlessness ⇒ Jan ash.

After

    Blister ⇒ Des gan.

    Weakness, intense ⇒ Caes bon.

Compound fever

Chill

    Alternate with sweat ⇒ Caes bon.

    Without ⇒ Term arj.

Heat, during

    Dyspnoea ⇒ Gent chi.

    Warm water desire for ⇒ Gent chi.

Without chill ⇒ Caes bon.

Sweat

    Profuse ⇒ Asai.

Bilious, bile excess with ⇒ Nyc arb.
Burning in whole body or in parts ⇒ Aza ind.
Chronic, weakness, seminal loss or gonorrhea due to ⇒ Tin cor.
Feeling ⇒ And pan. 10 gtt x tds (at).
Haematuria, with ⇒ Asai.
Malaria, Quinine abuse with ⇒ Aza ind.
Intense burning in whole body with ⇒ Old her.
Vertigo, cephalgia intense, with ⇒ Tric dio.

Gastritis

⇒ Car pap. 10 gtt 15 min before and after meals.
Burning in palm and sole, intense, with ⇒ Cep ind.
Cephalgia, with ⇒ Cep ind.

Helitosis

Infection due to ⇒ Gargle Term che. 15 gtt x tds. in warm water.

Impotency

Desire with ⇒ Fic rel.
Emission early ⇒ Oci grat. 10 gtt x tds., Oci rad.
Weakness, with ⇒ Fic ind., Hemi ind.
Induce to ⇒ Aeg fol.
Seminal deficiency with ⇒ With som. 20 gtt x tds.
Spermatorrhoea, with ⇒ Mor ind.

Lactation

Milk, increase to ⇒ Ric com.

Leucorrhoea ⇒ Wash with Are cat.

    Anaemia with, thin girls in ⇒ Abro rad.

    Chronic ⇒ Jan ash. 10 gtt x tds.

        Itching, with ⇒ Hemi ind.

            Externally washing the part with Jan ash. in ratio 1 : 9 provides good relief.

    Nymphomania, with ⇒ With som.

    Small, girls in ⇒ Can sat.

Lumbago

Intercourse, after ⇒ Can ind.

Mouth

Apthae, painful ⇒ Gargle with Term che. in ratio 1 : 4.

Dental plaques ⇒ Gargle with Are cat. in ratio 1 : 9

Helitosis ⇒ Gargle with Term che. in ratio 1 : 9.

Pyorrhoea ⇒ Gargle with Term che. in ratio 1 : 4.

Taste, wanting ⇒ Cas fis.

Ulcers ⇒ Gargle with Are cat. in ratio 1 : 4.

Menses

Breast pain, before ⇒ Agn cas.

Burning in body, menses before ⇒ Jan ash. 5 gtt x tds.

Discharges any form ⇒ Fic ind.
Induce to ⇒ Abro rad. 20 gtt x tds 4 – 5 dsys before expected menstrual period.
Irregular, cephalgia with ⇒ Jan ash. 5 gtt x tds.
    Sterility with ⇒ Jan ash. 5 gtt x tds.
Problem, hysteria with ⇒ Abro aug.
Painful ⇒ Car car.
    Cephalgia, with ⇒ Can ind.
    Nymphomania, with ⇒ Can ind.
    Profuse, with ⇒ Can ind.
    Scanty menses, with ⇒ Abro rad.
Profuse, Red, bloody ⇒ Fic rel.
    Menopause, during ⇒ Vis alb.
Suppressed
    Anaemia, with ⇒ Abro rad.
    Anasarca, due to ⇒ Cyn dac.
        Pain, with ⇒ Jan ash. 5 gtt x tds.
    Irritability, due to due to ⇒ Jan ash. 5 gtt x tds.
    Pain, due to ⇒ Jan ash.
    Weakness, due to ⇒ Jan ash. 5 gtt x tds.

Oedema

Anaemia, with ⇒ Just ad.
Anorexia, with ⇒ Boe diff. 10 gtt x tds (at).
General ⇒ Boe diff. 10 gtt x tds.
Heart problem, with ⇒ Aeg fol. 3 gtt x tds
Hepatomegaly, with ⇒ Luf bin.

Spleenomegaly, with ⇒ Luf bin.

Urination, promote to ⇒ Ach asp., Boe diff.

    Suppressed or scanty, with ⇒ Aeg fol.

Organ tonic

Blood ⇒ Tep pur.

Brain

    Cognition, to increase ⇒ Aco cal. 10 gtt x tds.

    Concentration, to increase ⇒ Aco cal.

    General ⇒ Bac mun. 10 gtt x tds.

Ear ⇒ Cit lim.

Gall bladder ⇒ Luf bin.

General

    Strength increase, to ⇒ Cyn dac. 3 gtt x od.

    Youth, maintain to ⇒ Emb off. 3 gtt x od.

Hair ⇒ Ecl alb. external application in ratio 1 : 4 (mix in pure coconut oil).

Heart ⇒ Term arj. 10 gtt x tds.

    Dyspnoea, with ⇒ Term bel.

Intestine ⇒ Emb rib.

Liver ⇒ Just ad.

    Infants, of ⇒ And pan.

Lungs ⇒ Lob in., Verb tha.

Nerves ⇒ Bac mun. 10 gtt x tds.

Kidneys ⇒ Tri ter. 10 gtt x tds.

Skin, Discolouration, skin disease after ⇒ Cal gig.

Spleen ⇒ Amoor roh., Heli an., Luf bin.

Tendon ⇒ Ana sat.

Uterus ⇒ Abro rad.

    Menses painful, with ⇒ Abro rad.

        Scanty, with ⇒ Abro aug.

Sexual desire

Increased, Palpitation with ⇒ Term arj.

Sleep

    Improper, Dreams, due to ⇒ Can ind.

    Frightful, due to ⇒ Term arj.

Sleeplessness

    Aged, in ⇒ Bac mun. 5 gtt x tds.

    Anxiety, with ⇒ Aco cal.

    Dysomnia ⇒ Abro aug.

    General ⇒ Hydr asia.

Sleep paralysis ⇒ With som. 10 gtt x tds.

Skin

Ailments, gastro intestinal problems, with ⇒ Crot t.

Gangrene ⇒ Calo gig.

Itching, Eruption, without ⇒ Aza ind.

    Burning, with ⇒ Cas sop. 10 gtt x tds.

Prickly heat ⇒ Aza ind.

    In upper part of the body ⇒ Syz jam.

Urticaria ⇒ Hygr spi.

Youthful, to maintain ⇒ With som. 5 gtt x od.

Stool

Has to go 2 – 3 times in morning, but passes little or no stool at times only air ⇒ Aeg mar. 20 gtt x tds.

Involuntary bloody stool ⇒ Tric dio.

Constipation

    Acidity, with ⇒ Nyc arb.

    Anurea, with ⇒ Can sat.

    Cephalgia, with ⇒ Emb off.

Diarrhea, followed by ⇒ Boe diff.

Dry stool, with ⇒ Abel mos.

Dyspnoea, with ⇒ Just ad.

Infants in ⇒ Emb off., Oci grat.

Liver problem, with ⇒ Aeg fol.

Malaria, after ⇒ And roh.

Diarrhoea

    Acute ⇒ Aeg mar. 20 gtt x horis.

        Pain in umbilical region, with ⇒ Cep ind.

            Whole abdomen, with ⇒ Hol ant. 10 gtt x tds (at).

    Anorexia, with ⇒ Cyp rot.

    Anurea, with ⇒ Asai.

        Chronic ⇒ Ric com.

Colic (which is not > stool) with ⇒ Atis ind.

Oedema, with ⇒ Cyn dac.

Cramp, before ⇒ Tric dio.

Dentitional, weakness, weight loss with ⇒ Sol nig. 7 gtt x tds x 10 days. (psk)

Dysentery

Amoebic ⇒ Atis rad.

Autumnal ⇒ Atis rad.

Bacillary ⇒ Atis rad.

Blood, navel pain, intense, with ⇒ Atis rad.

Pain in umbilical region, with ⇒ Cep ind.

Summers in ⇒ Hol ant. 15 gtt x horis.

Winter ⇒ Atis ind.

Malena ⇒ Asai.

Throat

Sore ⇒ Gargle Term che. 15 gtt x horis in luke warm water.

Voice, clear to make ⇒ Aco cal.

Tonsil

Follicular tonsillitis ⇒ Gargle Aza ind. 15 gtt x horis in luke warm water.

Inflammed ⇒ Gargle Term che. 15 gtt x horis in luke warm water.

Constipation, with ⇒ Term che. 10 gtt x tds.

Fever, after ⇒ Atis ind.

Urine

Incontinence of ⇒ Abro aug.
  Bed in ⇒ Blu od.
Nocturnal eneuresis, grinding of teeth with ⇒ Ver ant.
  Pot bellied, patients in ⇒ Emb rib.

Useful as

Anti cancerous agent ⇒ Bau var. 5 gtt x tds.
Birth control ⇒ Doli.
Broncho-dilator ⇒ Blat ori. 20 gtt as sos.
Detoxificant ⇒ And pan. 10 gtt x tds.
Diuretic ⇒ Boe diff. 15 gtt as sos.
Expectorant ⇒ Cal gig.
Haemostatic ⇒ Blu od. 20 gtt.
Hepato-protective ⇒ And pan. 10 gtt x tds.
Hepato-stimulative ⇒ And pan. 10 gtt x tds.
Nutritive ⇒ Tin cor. 10 gtt x tds.
Sudorific (Bring prespiration) ⇒ Psor cor.

Withdrawal effects of

Addiction any form ⇒ Aven sat. 20 gtt x tds.
Alcohol ⇒ Aven sat. 15 gtt x tds.
Asprin ⇒ Rau ser.
Opium ⇒ Aven sat. 20 gtt x tds.
Psychedelic drugs ⇒ Aco cal. 10 gtt x tds.
Tobacoo ⇒ Daph ind.

Worm

⇒ Cler inf.
Anorexia, with ⇒ Cyp rot.
Colic with ⇒ Atis ind.
Diarrhea with ⇒ Atis ind.
Frothy stool, with ⇒ Cler inf.
Gastritis, with ⇒ Atis ind., Emb rib.

Wound

Burst of pustule, after ⇒ And pan. 10 gtt x bd x 7 days. (psk).
Lacerated ⇒ Calen off. for external application in ratio 1 : 5.

REPERTORY OF INVESTIGATIONS

Blood
CBC
  Eosinophils
    Decrease to ⇒ Bac mun. 10 gtt x tds x 6 months.
  Haemoglobin
    Decrease to ⇒ Bac mun. 10 gtt x tds x 6 months.
      Bet vul. 15 gtt x tds x 3 months.
    Increase to ⇒ Hib.
  MCH
    Increase to ⇒ Bet vul. 15 gtt x tds x 3 months.
    Decrease to ⇒ Bac mun. 10 gtt x tds x 6 months.
  MCHC
    Decrease to ⇒ Bet vul. 15 gtt x tds x 3 months.
  MCV
    Increase to ⇒ Bac mun. 10 gtt x tds x 6 months.
      Bet vul. 15 gtt x tds x 3 months.
  PCV
    Decrease to ⇒ Aco cal. 10 gtt x tds x 3 months.
      Bac mun. 10 gtt x tds x 6 months.
      Bet vul. 15 gtt x tds x 3 months.

Platelets
    Increase to ⇒ With som.

RBC
    Decrease to ⇒ Bet vul. 15 gtt x tds x 3 months.
    Increase to ⇒ With som.

RDW
    Decrease to ⇒ Bac mun. 10 gtt x tds x 6 months.

Electrolytes ⇒ Alo ver., Nat mur bit.

ESR ⇒ Cler inf.

Glucose
    Increased, decrease to ⇒ Syz jam. 30 gtt x horis.
    Decreased, increased to ⇒ Bet vul. 15 gtt x tds.

Hormones
Gastrin
    Increase to ⇒ Cor sat.
Insulin
    Increase to ⇒ Jug reg.
Oestrogen
    Increase to ⇒ Foe vul.

Lipid profile ⇒ All sat., Are cat., Cal gig., Cor sat., Gly gla.
    Cholesterol, reduce to ⇒ Cur lon., Raph sat.

Fatty acid, reduce to ⇒ Emb off.
LDL, reduce to ⇒ Trac ammi.
Triglycerides, reduce to ⇒ Trac ammi.

LFT ⇒ And pan., Asaf., Car car., Cler inf., Pip nig.
    Bilirubin increased, quinine, abuse due to ⇒ Tin cor.
    Hepatomegaly with ⇒ And pan. 10 gtt x tds.
Alkaline Phosphatase
    Increase to ⇒ And pan. 10 gtt x tds.
    Decrease to ⇒ Aco cal. 10 gtt x tds x 3 months.
Bilirubin Direct ⇒ Leu as.
    Decrease to – Aco cal. 10 gt x tds x 3 months.
Globulin
    Increase to ⇒ And pan. 10 gtt x tds.
Total Protein
    Increase to ⇒ And pan. 10 gtt x tds.

RA Factor ⇒ Cler inf.

RFT ⇒ Arist ind., Oci bas.
Blood urea ⇒ Abel mos.
    Decrease to ⇒ Aco cal. 10 gtt x tds x 3 months.
Creatinine
    Decrease to ⇒ Tri ter. 15 gtt x tds.
Uric acid
    Decrease to ⇒ Aco cal. 10 gt x tds x 3 months.

Vitamin
- B – 1, deficient ⇒ Aeg fol.
- B – 2, deficient ⇒ Cor sat.
- C, deficient ⇒ Emb off, 10 gtt x tds x 3 months., Cit lim.

Blood poisoning ⇒ Hemi ind.

PFT ⇒ Aco cal., Amy am., Cat big., Crat nur., Hed hel, Ole San., Pip nig., Verb tha.
- Obstruction in bronchioles ⇒ Sass lap.

Semen ⇒ Agn cas., Arist ind., Oci bas., Ole san.
- Distorted shape ⇒ Jug reg.
- Increase, to ⇒ Psor cor.
- Polyzoospermia ⇒ Are cat.
- Thin ⇒ Mor ind.

Stool Test
C/E
- Occult blood ⇒ Blu od.

M/E
- Pus cells ⇒ San alb.
- RBC ⇒ Blu od.

P/E
- Colour, dark black ⇒ Heli an.

USG

Gall bladder

    Cholelithiasis ⇒ Raph sat.

Liver

    Hepatomegaly ⇒ And pan. 10 gtt x tds

        Chronic intermittent fever in ⇒ Leu as.

    Quinine, abuse due to ⇒ Tin cor.

    Spleenomegaly, chronic malaria, in ⇒ Aza ind., Caes bon.

Prostrate

    BHP, reduce to ⇒ Cuc pep.

Spleen

    Spleenomegaly

        Chronic intermittent fever in ⇒ Leu asp.

        Malaria, after ⇒ And roh.

        Quinine, abuse due to ⇒ Tin cor.

Urine examination ⇒ Ole San.

C/E

    Albumin ⇒ Abr aug. 10 gtt x tds x 3 months.

    Glucose, Higher, than corresponding blood glucose level ⇒ Syz jam.

    Ulcers at mouth of prepuce, causing ⇒ Abro aug.

    Occult blood ⇒ Blu od. 20 gtt x tds.

    Phosphates ⇒ Aven sat.

    Uric acid ⇒ Cocc cac., Oci can.

M/E
- RBC ⇒ Cyn dac 10 gtt x tds.
- Pus Cells ⇒ Oci grat.
- Sperm ⇒ Oci car.

P/E
- Appearance
  - Hazy ⇒ Crot t.
- Specific gravity
  - Increased ⇒ Gym syl.

CAUTION

This section contains the points which we should be cautious about while using a particular mother tincture. In general any mother tincture shall not be taken for more than 3 months continuously unless otherwise specified. After a gap of few weeks again it can be started.

Abelmoschus moschatus.

- Not to be used when patient is on Merformin, it is seen to hinder absorption of Metformin resulting in increase in blood glucose level.

Abroma augusta.

- It causes menses to appear, thereby not to be given during pregnancy.

Abrus precatorius.

- Not to be given in more than 5 gtt dose in children it causes harmful effects.
- In cases of uremia, avoid its use.

Achyranthes aspera.

- Avoid giving in thin people it reduces fat from abdomen and gluteal region.

Acorus calamus.

- Avoid using in renal failure cases, it increases glomerular damage.

- Avoid its use before and after surgery as it increases sleepiness. Stop taking it at least 2 weeks before scheduled surgery.

Agnus cas.

- It interferes with hormones so need not to be taken during lactation, menses, or pregnancy. Thereby it shall not be used in conditions that is hormone sensitive like – endometriosis, uterine fibroids, carcinoma of breast, ovaries and uterus.

- If patient is undergoing IVF, then better to avoid its use.

- Agnus cas effects dopamine secretion, so better to avoid it in cases of psychotic disorders like Schizophrenia.

Allium sativa.

- Not to be given to persons who suffer from any form of bleeding disorder or haemoglobinopathies.

Aloe vera.

- Not to be given in case of hypoglycemia.
- Its long term use effects heart.

Ammora rohituka.

- It reduces side effects of chemotherapy, so shall not be used in patients who are undergoing chemotherapy. Once it is over it can be used to improve his health and reduce the side effects.

Amygdala amara.

- Being rich is hydrocyanic acid, it depresses CNS. So, not to be used with sedatives or in person who is going to take anaesthesia for operative procedure.

Arctium lappa.

- It slows down the process of blood clotting, so avoid it in bleeding disorders and during surgery. If anyone is on Arctium lappa then he shall discontinue its use 2 weeks before date of operation.

Aristolochia indica.

- Anyone having family history of renal diseases or renal insufficiency then he shall not be given Aristolochia indica as it harms kidneys.

Averrhoa bilimbi.

- It is rich in Oxalic acid, so those having calcium oxalate calculi should not be given.

Azadirachta indica.

- When anyone has undergone organ transplant, he should not be given Azadirachta indica as it hampers the effect of medicines taken to prevent organ rejection.

Bacopa munneri.

- It increases calcium level in blood. So, it is wise to avoid it in those having calcium calculi.

Calotropis gigentea.

- It interferes with function of heart. So, anyone who is prone to heart diseases having increased level of homocystein or having some sort of heart disease shall not be given Calotropis gigentea.

Oleum ricini.

- Oleum ricini should not be given in cases of obstruction or narrowing of gut musculatures and in cases of inflammation of colon.

MODE OF PREPARATION OF HOMOEOPATHIC MOTHER TINCTURES OF PLANT KINGDOM

Systematic way of preparation of mother tincture is mentioned in pharmacopoeia; but, various pharmacopoeias have some difference in method of preparation. Different pharmaceuticals following different pharmacopoeia have different mode of preparation of drugs. As time passes with experience and for ease different pharmaceuticals carry on their own methods which they call "Trade Secret".

Composition of plant affects its medicinal properties and is dependent on its species and its natural environment. These specimens are usually collected in dry sunny weather, cleaned by careful shaking, brushing, and rinsing with distilled water. Some precautions needs to be taken like –

- Stem should be collected after the development of leaves.
- Barks are collected from young trees.
- Whole plant should be collected in flowering season partly in flower and partly in bud during sunny weather.
- Shrubs are collected before the sap arises.

Leaving apart these stuffs we find that Hahnemann has given instructions for preparing homoeopathic medicines from § 264 to § 271 in his Organon of Medicine. His instructions can be called as "Old method of preparation of drugs". These old methods we can still use to make mother tinctures of Indian medicines whose mother substance is available in our locality. Keeping this in mind to enable physician to prepare his own medicines, brief method of preparation is mentioned below.

Preparation depends on the sources, solubility and moisture content of the drug substance. Modes of preparation can be divided into four classes.

Class	Nature of Mother Substance
Class I	Highly juicy plant.
Class II	Medium juicy plant.
Class III	Least juicy plant.
Class IV	Dried vegetable plant or its parts

Class I –

This method is applicable for plants having large quantity of juice as mentioned under "Belladonna" in Materia Medica Pura.

Procedure –

- Take fresh plant or its parts like root, leaves, stem, fruit, etc. and cut it into small pieces.
- Grind it into pulp in grinder and express its juice by wringing the cloth.
- Immediately add an equal quantity by weight of strong alcohol to it before fermentation takes place in a jar.

- Shake it vigorously for few minutes and then keep it still for 8 days in cool dark place.

- The clear super-cumbent fluid is then decanted and filtered. This filtered extract is kept in clean amber brown glass bottle for use as mother tincture.

Class II –

This method is applicable for plants having medium quantity of juice as mentioned under "Thuja" in Materia Medica Pura. This is applied to non mucilaginous material containing resins, terpins and volatile oil.

Procedure –

- Take fresh plant or its parts like root, leaves, stem, fruit, etc. and cut it into small pieces.

- Grind it into pulp in grinder. Add 2 parts of strong alcohol to 3 part of pulp by weight in a jar.

- If pulp seems dry, more alcohol shall be added to moisten it, till the whole pulp is immersed in alcohol and kept for 3 days.

- Then the extract from the pulp is expressed out by wringing the cloth.

- Shake it vigorously for few minutes and then keep it still for 8 days in cool dark place.

- The clear super-cumbent fluid is then decanted and filtered. This filtered extract is kept in clean amber brown glass bottle for use as mother tincture.

Class III –

This method is applicable for plants having least quantity of juice.

Procedure –

- Take fresh plant or its parts like roots, leaves, stem, fruit, etc. and cut it into small pieces.

- Grind it into pulp in grinder. Add double part of alcohol to the pulp by weight in a jar.

- If pulp seems dry, more alcohol be added to moisten it, till the whole pulp is immersed in alcohol and kept for 3 days in a jar.

- Then the extract from the pulp is expressed out by wringing the cloth.

- Shake it vigorously for few minutes and then keep it still for 8 days in cool dark place.

- The clear super-cumbent fluid is then decanted and filtered. This filtered extract is kept in clean amber brown glass bottle for use as mother tincture.

Class IV –

This method of preparation is applicable for plants or its parts having least quantity of juice.

Procedure –

- Pulverize the dried mother substance into fine powder.

- Add 5 times strong alcohol to the weight of mother substance in a jar.

- Mix it and keep it in corked glass bottle for a fortnight in a dark place.

- Shake the mixture well twice a day.

- After a fortnight, decant the clear tincture, the residual substance is strained in new linen cloth and added to the previously decanted tincture.

- This is again filtered through filter paper and stored in glass corked bottle as mother tincture for further use.

Only the brief preparation of mother tinctures of herbs is mentioned to enable a physician to prepare his own mother tinctures by himself, when it is not available in market or none pharmaceuticals make it and its mother substance is present in abundance in his locality. If anyone wishes to know more about preparation of homoeopathic drugs, do refer to pharmacopoeia.

Generally one cannot prepare all the medicines for his use so he has to depend on pharmaceuticals. There are numerous pharmaceuticals, but I did not find a single company preparing all the mother tinctures which gives expected results always. Thereby, as practice taught me I use specific medicine of specific company. Giving list of those here will be tiresome and difficult, increasing the size of the book. So, anyone having queries and willing to know about these stuffs can mail me on drniteshhomoeopath@gmail.com.

LIST OF PLANTS WITH ITS PART USED FOR PREPARATION OF MOTHER TINCTURE

Sl.No.	List of Plants.	Parts used.
1.	Abroma augusta.	Leaf.
2.	Abroma radix.	Root.
3.	Abrus precatorius.	Seed.
4.	Acalypha indica.	Whole plant.
5.	Achyranthes aspera.	Leaf & Branch.
6.	Acorus calamus.	Dried root.
7.	Aegle folia.	Leaf.
8.	Aegle marmelos.	Fruit.
9.	Agnus cas.	Dried fruit.
10.	Allium cepa.	Fresh bulb.
11.	Allium sativa.	Fresh bulb.
12.	Aloe vera.	Juice from leaf.
13.	Amoora rohituka.	Bark.

Sl.No.	List of Plants.	Parts used.
14.	Amygdala amara.	Nut.
15.	Ananas sativa.	Stem & Juice.
16.	Andersonia rohitika.	Whole plant.
17.	Andrographis paniculata.	Whole plant.
18.	Arctium lappa.	Fresh root.
19.	Areca catechu.	Seed.
20.	Aristolochia indica.	Root.
21.	Asafoetida.	Gum.
22.	Atista indica.	Stem & leaf.
23.	Atista radix.	Root.
24.	Avena sativa.	Seed.
25.	Averrhoa bilimbi.	Fruit.
26.	Azadirachta indica.	Bark.
27.	Bacopa munneri.	Whole plant.
28.	Bauhinia variegate.	Bud.
29.	Beta vulgaris.	Root.
30.	Blumea odorata.	Whole plant.
31.	Boerhaavia diffusa.	Leaf & Root.
32.	Boerhaavia repens.	Seed.

Sl.No.	List of Plants.	Parts used.
33.	Bryophyllum calycinum.	Leaf.
34.	Caesalpinia bonducella.	Heart wood.
35.	Calendula officinalis.	Leaf.
36.	Calotropis gigentea.	Root.
37.	Cannabis indica.	Flower.
38.	Cannabis sativa.	Flower.
39.	Cantharanthus roseus.	Root & Shoot.
40.	Carica papaya.	Milk of papaya. (N. C. Ghosh)
41.	Carum carvi.	Seed.
42.	Cassia fistula.	Fruit.
43.	Cassia sophera.	Root.
44.	Catalpa bignonioides.	Bark.
45.	Cephalendra indica.	Leaf.
46.	Chrysopogon zizanioides.	Root.
47.	Cinnamonum.	Bark.
48.	Citrus limonum.	Juice.
49.	Clerodendron infortunatum.	Flower.
50.	Coleous aromaticus.	Leaf.

Sl.No.	List of Plants.	Parts used.
51.	Coriandrum sativum.	Leaves & Seed.
52.	Crateva nurvala.	Dried Bark.
53.	Crocus sativa.	Stigma of flower.
54.	Croton tig.	Seed.
55.	Cucurbita pepo.	Fruit.
56.	Cuminum cyminum.	Seed.
57.	Curcuma longa.	Rhizome.
58.	Cynodon dactylon.	Whole plant.
59.	Cyperus rotundus.	Tuber.
60.	Cyperus scariosus.	Tuber.
61.	Daphne indica.	Bark.
62.	Desmodium gangeticum.	Leaf.
63.	Daucus carota.	Fruit.
64.	Dolichos lablab.	Beans.
65.	Eclipta alba.	Leaf & Stem.
66.	Embelia officinalis.	Fruit.
67.	Embelia ribes.	Berries.
68.	Ficus benghalensis.	Bud.
69.	Ficus indica.	Root.

Sl.No.	List of Plants.	Parts used.
70.	Ficus religiosa.	Twig.
71.	Foeniculum vulgare.	Fruit.
72.	Genitsta tinctoria.	Flowering twig.
73.	Gentiana Chirata.	Whole plant.
74.	Glycyrrhiza glabra.	Root.
75.	Guggulu.	Gum resin.
76.	Gymnema sylvestre.	Whole plant.
77.	Gynocordia odorata.	Seed.
78.	Hedra helix.	Whole plant.
79.	Helianthus annus.	Seed.
80.	Hemidesmus indica.	Root.
81.	Hibiscus.	Flower.
82.	Holarrhena antidysentrica.	Bark & Seed.
83.	Hydrocotyle asiatica.	Whole plant.
84.	Hygrophila spinosa.	Whole plant
85.	Janosia ashoka.	Bark.
86.	Juglans regia.	Leaf.
87.	Justicea adhatoda.	Leaf.
88.	Justicea rubrum.	Flower.

Sl.No.	List of Plants.	Parts used.
89.	Leukas aspera.	Whole plant
90.	Lobelia inflata.	Whole plant.
91.	Luffa bindal.	Fruit.
92.	Mangifera indica.	Fruit.
93.	Menispernum.	Root.
94.	Morus indica.	Berries.
95.	Nardostachys grandiflora.	Rhizome.
96.	Nyctanthis arbortristis.	Leaf.
97.	Ocimum basilicum.	Leaf.
98.	Ocimum canum.	Leaf.
99.	Ocimum cariophylatum.	Leaf.
100.	Ocimum gratessium.	Leaf.
101.	Ocimum radix.	Root.
102.	Ocimum sanctum.	Leaf.
103.	Oldenlandia herbacea.	Flower.
104.	Oleum ricini.	Beans.
105.	Oleum santali.	Wood.
106.	Opuntia vulgaris.	Fruit.
107.	Phyllanthus niruri.	Fruit.

Sl.No.	List of Plants.	Parts used.
108.	Picrorhiza kurroa.	Rhizome.
109.	Piper nigrum.	Fruit.
110.	Psoralia corylifolia.	Seed.
111.	Rauvolfia serpentina.	Root.
112.	Raphanus sativa.	Root.
113.	Ricinus communis.	Leaf.
114.	Santalum album.	Heartwood.
115.	Sassurea lappa.	Rhizome.
116.	Semal.	Flower.
117.	Solonum nigrum.	Whole plant.
118.	Solanum xanthocarpus.	Root.
119.	Stellaria media.	Leaf.
120.	Syzygium jambolinum.	Seed.
121.	Tephrosia purpurea.	Whole plant.
122.	Terminalia arjuna.	Bark.
123.	Terminalia bellirica.	Fruit.
124.	Terminalia chebula.	Fruit.
125.	Tinospora cordifolia	Whole plant.
126.	Trachyspermum ammi.	Fruit & Seed.

Sl.No.	List of Plants.	Parts used.
127.	Tribulus terrestris.	Leaf & Shoot.
128.	Trichosanthes dioica	Fruit.
129.	Verbascum thapsus.	Flower & Leaf.
130.	Veronia anthelminthica.	Whole plant.
131.	Viola odorata.	Flower.
132.	Viola tricolor.	Whole plant.
133.	Viscum album.	Leaf.
134.	Withania somnifera.	Root.
135.	Withania somnifera folia.	Leaf & Stem.
136.	Withania somnifera rubra.	Flower.
137.	Wrightia tinctoria.	Whole plant.

LIST OF MEDICINES WITH THEIR COMMON NAMES IN SANSKRIT AND HINDI

Sl. No.	Scientific Name	संस्कृत नाम	हिंदी नाम
1.	Abelmoschus moschatus.	लताकस्तूरिका	मुश्कदाना, जंगली भिंडी
2.	Abroma augusta.	पिशाचकार्पास	उलटकम्बल
3.	Abrus precatorius.	गुन्जी	रति
4.	Acalypha indica.	हरितमंजरी	कुप्पी
5.	Achyranthes aspera.	अपामार्ग	चिरचिटा
6.	Acorus calamus.	वचा	घोरबच

Sl. No.	Scientific Name	संस्कृत नाम	हिंदी नाम
7.	Aegle folia.	बिल्वपत्र	बेलपत्ता
8.	Aegle marmelos.	कपित्थम्	बेलफल
9.	Agnus cas.	सिन्धुवार	निर्गुंडी
10.	Allium cepa.	सुकन्दक	प्याज
11.	Allium sativa.	लशुन	लहसुन
12.	Aloe vera.	गृहकन्या घृतकुमारी	ग्वारपाठा घीक्वार
13.	Amoora rohituka.	लक्ष्मी लोहिता	हरिनहरी
14.	Amygdala amara.		प्रमस्तिष्कखंड
15.	Ananas sativa.	अनानासम्	अनन्नास

Sl. No.	Scientific Name	संस्कृत नाम	हिंदी नाम
16.	Andersonia rohitika	रोहितक	रोहेड़ा
17.	Andrographis paniculata.	यवतिक्त भूनिम्ब महातिक्त	किरायत कालमेघ
18.	Areca catechu.	अकोट: चामरपुष्पु गुवाक:	चामरपुष्पु गुवाक सुपारी
19.	Aristolochia indica.	अर्कमूला ईश्वरी	ईश्वरमूल विषापहा
20.	Asafoetida.	हिङ्गु	हींग
21.	Atista indica.	आर्त्यशाखोट	वननिम्बु सरोहा

Sl. No.	Scientific Name	संस्कृत नाम	हिंदी नाम
22.	Avena sativa.	जयिन्	जई
23.	Averrhoa bilimbi.	कारमाराका अम्ल सिरालम्	बिलिम्बी
24.	Azadirachta indica.	निम्ब रविप्रिय	नीम
25.	Bacopa munneri.	ब्राह्मी निम्बलोणिका	नीरब्राह्मी सफेद चमनी
26.	Beta vulgaris.	पालङ्गशाक:	चुकंदर
27.	Blumea odorata.	कंकमर्दु कंकदर मट्टु छड़	जंगली मूली ककरम्भा

Sl. No.	Scientific Name	संस्कृत नाम	हिंदी नाम
28.	Boerhaavia diffusa.	पुनर्नवा	श्वेत पुनर्नवा
29.	Caesalpinia bonducella.	नादाकरञ्ज दुःस्पर्श गाडुम्बष्ठी	गजगा कलिंग करंज
30.	Calendula officinalis.	जेरगुल	गेंदा
31.	Calotropis gigentea.	मन्दार अर्क कहिव:	सफेद आक मदार
32.	Cannabis indica.	भांग	भांग
33.	Cantharanthus roseus.	सदाफूली	सदाबहार

Sl. No.	Scientific Name	संस्कृत नाम	हिंदी नाम
34.	Carica papaya.	पारिश	पपीता, पोपया
35.	Carum carvi.	कारवी	कृष्णजीर:
36.	Cassia fistula.	आरग्वधः, राजवृक्षः, शम्पाकः, चतुरङ्गुलः	अमलतास
37.	Cassia sophera.	कासमर्दै	कसौंदी, बासकी
38.	Cephalendra indica.	बिम्ब, बिम्बीफल	कन्दूरी

Sl. No.	Scientific Name	संस्कृत नाम	हिंदी नाम
39.	Chrysopogon zizanioides.	अभया अमरीनाता	खस
40.	Cinnamonum.	दारुसिता वराङ्गम्	दालचीनी
41.	Citrus limonum.	निम्बूकः	निम्बू
42.	Clerodendron infortunatum.	घण्टक भाण्डिर	भाण्टा घण्टाकर्ण
43.	Coleous aromaticus.	पाषाणभेदी हिमसागर	पत्थरचूर आमरोडा
44.	Coriandrum sativum.	कस्तुम्बरी	धनिया
45.	Crateva nurvala.	वरण	बरना

Sl. No.	Scientific Name	संस्कृत नाम	हिंदी नाम
46.	Crocus sativa.	कश्मीरजन्मन्	केसर
47.	Croton tig.	निम्बडीफलम्	जमालघोटा
48.	Cucurbita pepo.	कर्कटिः	सफेद कद्दू कुम्हड़ा
49.	Curcuma longa.	हरिद्रा	हल्दी
50.	Cynodon dactylon.	सहस्रवीर्य अनंत भार्गवी	दूब दूर्वा
51.	Cyperus scariosus.	नागरमुस्तक भद्र मुस्तक	बड़ा नागर मोथा कोरैही झाड़

Sl. No.	Scientific Name	संस्कृत नाम	हिंदी नाम
52.	Desmodium gangeticum.	अंशुमती ध्रुवा दीर्घमूला पीवरी	शालपर्णी सालपानी पीवरी शारीबान
53.	Dolichos lablab.	निष्पाव	सेम
54.	Eclipta alba.	भिंगराज	केशराज
55.	Embelia officinalis.	आमलकी	आँवला
56.	Embelia ribes.	आम्रेय:	बायबिड़ंग
57.	Ficus indica.	वट	बड़
58.	Ficus religiosa.	श्रीवृक्ष	पीपल

Sl. No.	Scientific Name	संस्कृत नाम	हिंदी नाम
59.	Foeniculum vulgare.	मिसरेया मधुरिका	मोटी सौंफ
60.	Gentiana chirata.	किरातितिक्तं अनार्यतिक्तं	चिरायता नीलकान्त
61.	Glycyrrhiza glabra.	जलयष्टि	मुलहठी
62.	Guggulu.	गुग्गुलु	गुग्गुलु
63.	Gymnema sylvestre.	मेषशृङ्गी	गुड़मार
64.	Gynocordia odorata.	पाटली	चालमुंगरा
65.	Helianthus annus.	सूर्यविन्	सूरजमुखी
66.	Hemidesmus indica.	अनन्तमूल्	कलीसार

Sl. No.	Scientific Name	संस्कृत नाम	हिंदी नाम
67.	Hibiscus.	जपाठ	गुरहल
68.	Holarrhena antidysenterica.	कुटज इन्द्रजव	कुरैया कुटर्ची
69.	Hydrocotyle asiatica.	मण्डूकपर्णी	बेंगुकी
70.	Hygrophila spinosa.	कोकिलाक्ष क्षुरक	
71.	Janosia ashoka.	अशोक	अशोक
72.	Juglans regia.	अखोड़ा	अखरोट
73.	Justicea adhatoda.	बासक सिंहमुखी	अडूसा रास

Sl. No.	Scientific Name	संस्कृत नाम	हिंदी नाम
74.	Leucas aspera.	द्रोणपुष्पी चित्रपत्रिका	गुम्मा गुमामधुपति
75.	Lobelia inflata.	मिरिपुष्य	धवल तम्बाखू
76.	Luffa bindal.	कोशातकी देवदाली	बिन्दल घागोर बेल
77.	Mangifera indica.	आम्रम	आम
78.	Morus indica.	तूत	शहतूत
79.	Nardostachys grandiflora.	जटामानसी	जटामानसी
80.	Nyctanthis arbortristis.	पारिजात शेफालिका	हर हरशिंगार

Sl. No.	Scientific Name	संस्कृत नाम	हिंदी नाम
81.	Ocimum basilicum.	बर्बुरी	राम तुलसी
82.	Ocimum canum.	गरमिरा	श्याम तुलसी
83.	Ocimum cariophylatum.	मंजरिकी	दुलाल तुलसी
84.	Ocimum gratessium.	अजका फणिज्जक	बन तुलसी मरुवा
85.	Ocimum sanctum.	विष्णुप्रिया	काली तुलसी
86.	Oldenlandia herbacea.	पर्पट	पित्तपापड़ा
87.	Phyllanthus niruri.	भूम्यामलकी	भूमी आंवला
88.	Picrorhiza kurroa.	कटम्भरा	करड़ी
89.	Piper nigrum.	मरिच	काली मिर्च

Sl. No.	Scientific Name	संस्कृत नाम	हिंदी नाम
90.	Psoralia corylifolia.	वकुची	बावची
91.	Raoulfia serpentine.	चन्द्रिका	सर्पगन्धा
92.	Raphanu ssativa.	मूलक	मूली
93.	Ricinus communis.	एरण्ड	अरंडी
94.	Santalum album.	अग्निदिता	चंदन
95.	Saussurea lappa.	पुष्कर कुष्ठ	कुट पोखरमूल
96.	Solonum nigrum.	स्वर्णक्षीरी	मकोय
97.	Solanum xanthocarpus.	कण्टकारी	भटकटैया
98.	Syzygium jambolanum.	नीलफल	जामुन

Sl. No.	Scientific Name	संस्कृत नाम	हिंदी नाम
99.	Terminalia arjuna.	अर्जुन	अर्जुन
100.	Terminalia bellirica.	अक्ष	बहेड़ा
101.	Terminalia chebula.	हरीतकी	हड़
102.	Tinospora cordifolia.	गुडूची	गुरुच
103.	Trachyspermum ammi.	अजमोद	अजवाईन
104.	Tribulus terrestris.	अश्वदंष्ट्रा	गोखुरु
105.	Trichosanthes dioica.	पटोल	परवल
106.	Tylophora indica.	अर्कपर्णि	जंगलिपिकवान
107.	Veronia anthelmintica.	सोमराज	सोमराज
108.	Withania coagulans.	रिश्यगंधा	पनीरफूल

Sl. No.	Scientific Name	संस्कृत नाम	हिंदी नाम
109.	Withania somnifera.	बलदा	अश्वगंधा
110.	Wrightia tinctoria.	बाजीकरी	कघार

* Numerous names could not be confirmed so they are not added in the list.

www.ingramcontent.com/pod-product-compliance
Lightning Source LLC
Chambersburg PA
CBHW030915180526
45163CB00004B/1846